INTRODUCTION

Pimples are hard and inflamed spots on the skin. They originate in the follicles when dead skin cells mix with excess oil, causing bacteria to grow and clog the pores. Pimples typically form on your face, neck, back, chest, or shoulders and can appear at any age. Although pimples are common, the effects go beyond the skin's surface.

Research has found that pimples are a common occurrence among teens. However, acne can also occur in adults and is commonly called adult acne. It is similar to teenage acne, as the factors causing teenage acne are the same as those present in adult acne.

Adult acne can be more persistent than the teenage version as it is often a continuation or relapse from adolescence. However, those who have never been affected by acne can also experience this.

There is not enough concrete evidence to suggest that what we eat is directly responsible for pimples. However, there may be some links between pimple formation and diets with a high glycemic index (GI) (these are highly processed foods that rapidly raise blood sugar). Proteins in dairy and milk products can also contribute to acne development.

A 2021 review found that certain vitamins and minerals may help reduce inflammation caused by acne. These include vitamins A, C, E, zinc, and selenium. While these results were promising, the conclusions were not definitive and only suggest that nutrition may be one of many contributing factors in pimple formation.

If you suspect that certain dietary changes may be responsible for your pimples, it is best to speak to a doctor or board-certified dermatologist about this before making any changes. They may suggest keeping a food diary to log your meals and any changes that may result from eating certain foods.

While no one gene causes acne, some research indicates that genetics can influence how severe your pimples are. Several studies have found that people with a family history of acne were more likely to experience it in their lifetime.

In a separate study examining the genetic makeup of 20 identical and non-identical twins, researchers noted that sebum control also appeared to be influenced by genetic factors. Those with oily skin types showed an increased risk of acne because it is an ideal environment for acne-causing bacteria to grow.

There is a range of treatments that can reduce the spread of pimples to other parts of your body, such as applying a warm, damp towel to the pimple could help bring the pus and excess sebum closer to the surface of your skin. However, it is best not to squeeze or push down on the pimple once this has happened, as this could cause more inflammation and possibly move the infected content further into the skin, both leading to a greater chance of scarring.

If your skin is relatively clear with the occasional pimple, spot treatments may be enough. These are targeted solutions in the form of patches, drying lotions, or creams that you can apply to your pimple. What makes these spot treatments so effective are their ingredients, which typically include nonprescription components such as benzoyl peroxide, salicylic acid, and sulfur.

Nonprescription OTC medications are common quick-fix treatments, including benzoyl peroxide, salicylic acid, and vitamin A derivatives (retinoids). These products come in many forms but ultimately treat pimples by reducing inflammation and killing the bacteria, or slowing its growth. At the same time, these products assist in removing dead skin cells and sebum and may help prevent pimples from returning.

These OTC products will often help clear pimples in six weeks or less. However, it is important to note that OTC medications do not have an obvious effect until you've used them every day for several weeks to a month.

If OTC medications are not helping, it may be time to consider prescription medicines. Prescription-strength medicines include oral and topical antibiotics, oral and topical retinoids, and hormone-based medication. These medications can kill acne-causing bacteria, normalize the shedding of dead skin cells, keep pores clear, and reduce the number of comedones. The doctor or dermatologist prescribing these medications will help create the best treatment plan for your lifestyle and medical history.

Pimples are not entirely avoidable, but there are several things you can do to help reduce them forming. Avoid touching your face to prevent the spread of dirt and bacteria, Practice good skincare habits with suitable products to prevent further breakouts, Avoid scratching or popping pimples to lessen the risk of infection and scarring, Avoid tight clothing so as not to irritate the pimples on your shoulders or back, Change your bed sheets regularly, Avoid using makeup around the affected area and Avoid excessive scrubbing of skin to prevent the opening of wounds.

CHAPTER ONE

WHAT ARE PIMPLES

Pimples are clogged pores (hair follicles) that have become inflamed. They're generally the result of the overproduction of oil in your skin combined with bacteria.

You're most likely to get pimples in areas with a lot of oil glands, which includes your face, neck, shoulders, chest, and back. Common types of inflamed pimples include papules, pustules, nodules, and cysts.

Acne comes in several types, depending on the types of pimples it causes. Knowing which type you have can help you choose the best treatment for your skin.

All pimples begin as a pore blockage or comedo. At first, a pimple is a small bump that isn't inflamed. A comedo becomes inflamed when bacteria infect it. This can also happen when it's irritated by squeezing. An inflamed pimple is red and swollen. Different types of pimples respond to different medications. Certain types of acne may require specialized treatment.

4 TYPES OF PIMPLES AND HOW TO TREAT THEM

Papules

Papules is inflamed blemishes. They appear on the skin's surface. They look like red bumps or lumps on the skin. They don't have a white head. Papules can be large or small. They can occur anywhere on the face or body, including your:

• Neck

• Chest

• Shoulders

• Back

• Buttocks

Causes: Papules can be caused by acne vulgaris. This occurs when the wall of a hair follicle ruptures. Hair follicles are also called pores.

When this happens, cellular debris and bacteria spill into the dermis. The dermis is the deepest layer of skin. A break in the pore can occur when the follicle fills with dead skin cells and oil. Pressure from squeezing a blackhead or blocked pore can also cause a rupture.

The rupture triggers inflammation in and around the follicle. The area turns red and swells. This is what creates the firm red bump we call a pimple.

Treatment: Don't squeeze a papule to try and make it come to a head. You probably won't extract any debris from the pore. Instead, you may simply make it more inflamed.

Papules are not deep lesions. This means most of them will heal quickly without scarring. Over-the-counter (OTC) benzoyl peroxide treatments can help heal acne papules. They may also prevent new blemishes from forming. If OTC products don't improve your breakouts after 10 to 12 weeks, though, you may need a prescription acne medication.

Pustules

Pustules are red and inflamed with an obvious head. The head is often white. That's why these blemishes are also called whiteheads. The head can also be cream to yellow in color.

Sometimes a brownish spot appears in the middle of the head. This is the comedonal core. It is a plug of debris within the pore. Acne pustules range in size from small to fairly large. They develop in the same areas that papules do. This is usually the face, back, and shoulders.

Causes: Pustules follow papules. When the pore ruptures, the body sends white blood cells to fight bacteria. This is what causes pus.

A mixture of pus, dead skin cells, and excess oil gives a pustule its white cap. Squeezing a pimple extracts this material. Popping pimples is never a good idea. When you squeeze a pimple you can drive the contents deeper into the pore. This can make the blemish much worse.

Treatment: Mild acne or occasional pustules can be treated at home with OTC benzoyl peroxide creams or cleansers. Acne spot treatments containing salicylic acid can also help.

See a dermatologist if:

• You have many pustules

• Your pustules are very inflamed

• Your acne is hard to control with OTC products

Prescription medications like topical retinoids or combination acne treatments can help.

Nodules

Nodules are serious acne pimples. They are large, inflamed lesions. They feel like hard, painful lumps under the skin. Papules and pustules occur at the surface, but nodules form deeper within the skin.

Causes: An acne nodule develops when the follicle wall ruptures deep within the dermis. Contaminated debris from the follicle infects nearby follicles.

The damage and Irritation causes the area to swell. This makes nodules quite painful. Like pustules, nodules can be filled with pus. Because they occur deep within the skin, though, you won't see a white head.

Females are prone to getting acne nodules around the time of their monthly cycle.

What Is Hormonal Acne? Hormonal acne is acne that affects adults between ages 20 and 50. It is caused when hormones cause an excess of sebum in oil glands. While it can affect any gender, it is more common in women and can be linked to menstrual cycles, pregnancy, and menopause.

Treatment: Occasional nodules can usually be treated at home. If your blemish is painful, you can ice the area to help relieve swelling. Don't try squeezing a nodule or any other pimple.

Nodules can take between a few weeks and several months to fully heal. This is because they are large and deep. Ask your dermatologist about a cortisone injection. This can help make your pimples go away faster.

If you're prone to nodular breakouts, you'll definitely want to make an appointment with a dermatologist. These types of blemishes don't respond to over-the-counter acne treatments. You'll need a prescription acne medication to get them under control.

Cysts

Cysts are very large, inflamed lesions. They feel like soft, fluid-filled lumps under the skin. Acne cysts are the most severe form of pimple. They can be very painful.

Causes: Like nodules, cysts begin as a deep break in the follicle wall. The body tries to wall off the infection by surrounding it with a membrane.

As an acne cyst works its way to the surface, it damages healthy skin tissue. This can destroy the follicle. The likelihood of acne scarring is very high. An acne cyst isn't a true cyst. It is actually a severe, swollen, acne nodule. You may hear the terms acne cyst and acne nodule used interchangeably.

Acne cysts are filled with pus. They may also contain blood. They can take several weeks to several months to fully heal. Never try to extract an acne cyst on your own. If they must be drained, it has to be done by a doctor.

Treatment: If you are prone to cystic acne, talk to a dermatologist. OTC acne treatments won't help these blemishes. There are no home remedies that can successfully treat cystic acne.

Oral acne medications like Absorica (isotretinoin) are the best treatment options for cystic acne. Cystic breakouts scar easily. The sooner you see a dermatologist about your acne, the sooner you will see improvement.

CAUSES OF PIMPLE

Here are some of the major causes of pimples:

• Excessive oil production by the sebaceous glands can lead to pores getting clogged by dirt and dead skin cells, causing acne and pus-filled pimples.

• Bacterial infections are caused by a certain kind of bacteria called P. acnes which lives at the base of the hair follicle and leads to the development of breakouts.

• Skin inflammation is a defensive response of your body towards both external and internal aggressors like allergies and other infections. It is the major cause of many skin issues, including pimples and breakouts.

• Certain dietary staples, like aerated drinks, white bread, white rice, and processed sugar can lead to breakouts and pimples. This is because the carbohydrates in these foods raise the glycemic index in your body and disturb the blood sugar levels.

• If your skin is overly sensitive to the testosterone hormone, it results in excessive sebum production. This, in turn, leads to increased hormonal acne and breakouts, more in some people as compared to others.

CHAPTER TWO

HOW TO GET RID OF PIMPLES FAST

Pimples always seem to pop up at the most inopportune times: just before prom night, the day before your wedding, or the morning of that important job interview. Breakouts are never welcomed, but it's times like these when you really want to get rid of pimples fast.

While they won't prevent acne from occurring, these quick fixes can help banish individual blemishes when you need to heal that pimple fast.

Use an Acne Spot Treatment

Over-the-counter (OTC) acne spot treatments are a good go-to when you have an inconvenient blemish. They're inexpensive, and you can buy them any store in the skin care aisle.

Dab a small amount of spot treatment directly onto the pimple. Some spot treatments are made to be left on overnight. Others are incorporated into a makeup concealer or are tinted to help conceal the blemish while it heals.

The most effective spot treatments contain either benzoyl peroxide or salicylic acid. Experiment to find which works best for you.

If you'd rather go the all-natural route, try dabbing on a drop of tea tree essential oil once or twice a day, or buy a spot treatment that contains tea tree. Although it hasn't been proven, some research shows tea tree oil may help treat acne breakouts.

Some people are sensitive to tea tree oil. Be cautious until you know how your skin will react and stop using if your skin gets irritated.

No matter what type of spot treatment you use, read the directions for that particular product and follow them. Even though it's tempting, don't apply more often than recommended. You'll wind up with flaky, irritated skin.

Although things like toothpaste, cinnamon, lemon, or the like are sometimes recommended as home remedies for pimples, there is no evidence that they actually work. They can also cause contact dermatitis (a rash caused by skin-irritating substances), so it's wise to stay away from them especially if you have sensitive skin.

Spot treatments work best on minor blemishes. They are not effective for serious breakouts like acne nodules and acne cysts.

Apply a Sulfur Mask

If spot treatments aren't quite helping, you may have better luck with a sulfur mask. Sulfur helps unclog pores and reduce inflammation, so it can help that swollen pimple look smaller.

Sulfur has been used as an acne treatment for many years. Today's treatments don't have the unpleasant scent of those from years past, luckily.

You can apply the mask on just the offending pimple or over the entire face (this has the added benefit of making large pores appear smaller.) Facial masks containing sulfur can be found at the drug store, department stores, or salons.

Some products can be left on as spot overnight treatment for maximum effectiveness; others must be rinsed off after a few minutes. Make sure you follow the directions on your product, and never leave a mask on overnight unless it specifically says it's OK to do so.

Ice It Down

Here's a trick often employed by estheticians. Apply an ice cube to inflamed blemishes to help reduce redness, swelling, and pain. This is also a cool fix for those blemishes you can't yet see but can feel as a sore lump under the skin.

You never want the ice cube directly touching your skin, so first wrap it in a soft cloth. Don't ice the pimple for too long (frostbite anyone?) Ice for 20 or 30 seconds, followed by a minute or so of rest, a few times per day or just before you go out.

Why icy cold and not hot? If you're trying to hide a pimple or reduce its size, the worst thing you could do is steam it or apply a hot compress just before you go out. Heat expands, so it will make the pimple look larger and redder.

This is one tip that you can use for both minor blemishes and more severe inflamed pimples, like nodules and acne cysts. Icing won't make the blemish heal faster, but it can definitely ease the pain of these swollen breakouts.

Get a Cortisone Injection

For those incredibly deep, painful zits and cystic breakouts that don't want to heal, a cortisone injection may be an option for you. During this quick procedure, a diluted cortisone is injected into the blemish.

Within just a few hours, the swelling will recede and the pain will go away. The breakout completely flattens out within 48 hours generally.

Large, deep blemishes usually don't respond well to other treatments, so if you absolutely need that breakout gone quickly a cortisone shot is your best bet. Ideally, you'll want to talk to your healthcare provider about this option before you really need one.

Cortisone injections aren't meant to be used as a regular treatment for big zits, but they're helpful in some cases and when used judiciously.

Stop Breakouts Before They Start

These tips are helpful for treating individual pimples, but if you're constantly battling acne the ultimate goal is to stop pimples from forming in the first place. For this, you'll need to use a good acne medication daily.

Over-the-counter products can work for mild acne. If your acne is inflamed, stubborn, and especially if you have severe acne or nodular breakouts, you'll need a prescription medication.

Don't hesitate to give your dermatologist a call. Your dermatologist can help devise an acne treatment plan to clear your skin.

HOW TO REMOVE PIMPLES AT HOME

Now that you are familiar with the causes of pimples, here are some natural ways of getting rid of them at home. Do make sure to not overdo these home remedies and always do a patch test before applying any kitchen ingredient on your face.

Turn to aloe vera and garlic paste

Aloe vera is an excellent hydrating agent for the skin and combined with the antiseptic and clarifying properties of garlic, can be a good detox mask for curing pimples. Allicin, an active compound found in garlic is anti-bacterial in nature. When combined with the antioxidant properties of aloe vera, they fasten healing and help treat pimples.

How to use: Crush two cloves of peeled garlic to form a paste. Add the 1 teaspoon of fresh aloe vera pulp to it and mix thoroughly. Apply the mixture on the affected area, leave it for 20 minutes and wash it off with warm water. Repeat this once a day until the pimple subsides.

Banana Peel

After you've gobbled down a banana, don't throw away the peel! We say that because bananas are rich in potassium, vitamins, and minerals; many of which are stored in the peel. It is this nourishing group of nutrients that will help strengthen the barrier of your skin and protect it from damage and breakouts.

How to use: Cut out a small portion of a ripe banana peel and place the inner white side over your skin. Rub it gently for 10 minutes and wash your face. Repeat this twice a day and within a couple of days, you can say goodbye to pimples!

If you're wondering how to reduce pimples at home, turn to the trusted combination of cinnamon and honey. Thanks to the anti-inflammatory properties of cinnamon and anti-bacterial honey, your pimples will soon be non-existent.

How to use: Combine ½ teaspoon of cinnamon with 2 tablespoons of honey to create a thick paste. Apply it all over the affected area and leave it for 30 minutes. Wash it off with warm water and repeat the treatment once a day.

Ice it away

A surprising yet effective method to get rid of pimples is using ice cubes. The temperature of the ice cube constricts the blood vessels beneath the surface of the skin, which reduces its size.

How to use: Place a single ice cube directly on top of a pimple and keep it there for about 3 minutes. Repeat the method twice a day until your pimple is gone.

Opt for baking soda

The next time a zit troubles you, remember that baking soda isn't just for cakes. With its excellent exfoliating powers, baking powers strips away oily residue, balances the pH level of the skin and eases irritation.

How to use: Gently rub a paste of baking powder and water directly on your pimple and leave it for 10 minutes. Wash it away thoroughly and repeat it every alternate day.

Use apple cider vinegar

Raw apple cider vinegar has been known to contain acetic, citric, lactic and succinic acid, all of which are capable of killing acne-causing bacteria on your face.

How to use: Dilute some raw ACV with water in the concentration of 1:3. Wash your face with a mild cleanser then apply the ACV solution on your pimples with a cotton ball, let sit for 5-10 minutes and wash with cold water. Follow up with a moisturiser and repeat everyday week for best results.

Tea tree oil is one of the most popular spot treatments that is used for acne. Combining its anti-inflammatory and antimicrobial properties, this essential oil can help reduce the size of acne lesions and cure them in a gentle way. But make sure to check you are not sensitive to the essential oil before applying it on your face.

How to use: Mix 1-2 drops of tea tree oil with 10-12 drops of jojoba carrier oil. Wash your face with a gentle cleanser and pat dry. Spot treat with the diluted oil just on your pimples with a Q-tip. Allow it to dry and follow up with your regular moisturiser. Do this twice a day for best results.

Tone your skin with witch hazel extract

Witch hazel is a natural astringent and has been used in skincare remedies for ages. When it comes to pimples, witch hazel can dry out blemishes and clear blackheads and whiteheads from your pores too.

How to use: Take a couple of drops of witch hazel toner on a cotton pad and apply all over your face. Do this every day after cleansing your face and follow up with a moisturiser to avoid over-drying your face.

Use green tea to soothe inflammation

Infused with the antioxidant compound called epigallocatechin-3-gallate (EGCG), helps regulate sebum production, fight inflammation and inhibit the growth of acne-causing bacteria in your skin.

How to use: Spritz some water on a couple of tea bags and put them in the fridge. When the tea bags are nice a cold, plop them on your blemishes and keep for about 10 minutes. Wash off with cold water and repeat any number of times you want throughout the day.

CHAPTER THREE

IS POPPING PIMPLES BAD FOR YOUR SKIN?

Popping pimples can be very tempting, but resist the urge. When you pop a pimple, it damages the underlying tissue and can leave your complexion looking worse.

Popping pimples on your face, back, chest, or buttocks can lead to more breakouts, discoloration, and acne scars.

Pimples and Inflammation

We've been warned by our dermatologists, estheticians, and even our mothers—do not pop pimples. Yes, popping pimples is as bad for our skin as the experts say.

A pimple occurs when excess sebum (oil), dead skin cells, and bacteria become trapped in a pore. This leads to the development of red, tender bumps with white pus at their tips.

When you have a pimple, the pore is already swollen and under a lot of pressure.

While your instinct may be to squeeze a pimple, consider what is happening under the skin.

When you squeeze a pimple:

a. You can force the debris from the pore deeper into the follicle (the structure that anchors each strand of hair to the skin).

b. That can cause the follicle wall to rupture, spilling the infected material (including pus) into the lower layer of skin, called the dermis.

c. This can result in even more inflammation than before, with increased redness, swelling, and heat in the surrounding skin.

d. The break in the structure of the skin can also promote infection, which can, in turn, lead to the formation of an even larger pimple and/or a new pimple right next to the one you just popped.

Have you ever popped a pimple thinking you "got" it, only to have it come back a few hours later bigger and "angrier" than before? You're not imagining things. That's because the damage happens below the surface of the skin and on the surface as well.

How the Skin Changes After You Pop a Pimple

In addition to new pimples forming near a pimple that's been squeezed, other skin changes, such as scars, and discoloration, can occur too.

Popping a papule (a pimple without a white head) forces the skin to break open to release the pus. This leads to the formation of a scab and the darkening of the surrounding skin.

Squeezing the area frequently can lead to the formation of acne nodules (hardened acne lesions in deeper tissues) or acne cysts (deep, pus-filled lesions that look similar to boils).

Popping pimples can cause more than a swollen spot or a scab; it is a surefire way to increase your chances of developing acne scars.

Every time your skin is damaged, there's a possibility tissue will be lost during the healing process. That is how you get depressed or pitted acne scars. The more extensive the damage, the higher the chance of tissue loss.

Even if depressed scars don't develop, you can be left with dark marks known as post-inflammatory hyperpigmentation. This occurs when severe inflammation damages cells known as keratinocytes, causing them to release large amounts of a pigment called melanin.

If the damage is minimal, the darkening of the skin will often reverse. But, if the damage is severe or ongoing, the discoloration may lighten but not entirely disappear without treatment.

Picking at pimples can spread infection and worsen your acne. Clearly, a "hands-off" policy is the best choice when it comes to caring for acne-prone skin.

With that said, it's natural to want to get rid of pimples and get rid of them fast. Fortunately, there are safer ways to do so.

Acne Spot Treatments

Instead of popping a pimple, try over-the-counter (OTC) acne spot treatments. These products are dabbed on existing pimples to help them dry and heal. These include products containing benzoyl peroxide, salicylic acid, or sulfur. You can also try a warm compress or hydrocolloid pimple bandaids to help shrink a pimple that's bothering you.

These OTC remedies work best for relatively minor pimples. You may need to see a dermatologist if you have a really big pimple that won't go away. Spot treatments are unlikely to be of much help with more severe blemishes.

Safer Blemish Extractions

When considering how to manage acne breakouts, it's important to understand that some options are safe, some are not ideal but are likely harmless, and some could be dangerous or unhealthy.

At one point or another, most people have popped a pimple even though they knew they shouldn't. Occasionally squeezing a blemish, while not great for your skin, is normal and understandable.

But, when squeezing pimples becomes a compulsion, you may develop a condition known as acne excoriée (or excoriated acne). People with excoriated acne pick at their pimples, real or imagined, to the point of seriously damaging their skin. You can learn to stop this behavior, but you will likely need the help of a professional, particularly if acne is causing ongoing anxiety or depression.

You may consider booking an appointment with a dermatologist or esthetician experienced in professional pimple extraction. They may teach you how to pop a pimple safely and how to decide whether it's safe for you to pop a pimple at home.

Among some of the things you should never do when popping pimples:

a. Never use your fingernails or another hard object to squeeze a pimple.

b. Never force a pimple to pop.

c. Never pop a pimple that doesn't have a white or yellow "head."

Popping a pimple is something you should make every effort to avoid. Doing so can force the contents of the pimple into deeper tissues. This can lead to skin inflammation, the formation of new pimples in nearby areas, scarring, and discoloration. In some cases, the damage caused to the skin may be permanent.

Instead of popping pimples, try over-the-counter acne medications or seek professional pimple extraction by a dermatologist or esthetician. If you can't resist popping a pimple, ask your dermatologist how to do so. Severe acne often requires treatment by a doctor.

HOW TO POP A PIMPLE AND EXTRACT A BLACKHEAD

You're likely to want to pop a pimple at some point, though there are safer and smarter ways to deal with your skin blemishes.

If that's the case, then you'll want to know how to do it without causing more skin damage. You'll also want to avoid infection, especially if something more than a pimple is going on with your skin.

Why You Should Avoid Popping Pimples

Hands down, the safest thing for your skin is "hands-off." The best way to deal with your pimple is to allow it to heal naturally. In other words, you should avoid popping or squeezing it.

If you do squeeze a pimple, you may be able to drain some pus from it. The problem is that the squeeze pushes the pimple both up and down. It's not just the pus that you're moving, either. The pimple's core holds a plug of dead skin cells and sebum, a natural kind of oil.

When you squeeze your pimple, you push this plug further into the affected skin pore. The pressure from the popping also may cause the wall of the pore to burst. This happens below the skin surface where you can't see it and means the infection can spread in the dermis layer of the skin.

That's why popping a pimple can cause more damage than just leaving it alone. The more the skin is damaged, the higher the chance you may develop acne scarring.

It's best to let a pimple heal by itself. That's because popping or squeezing a pimple won't just remove the pus you see. It also pushes it into the nearby skin. This spreads the infected matter and can cause more skin damage.

Solutions Without Popping

There are other ways to get a pimple to drain without popping. Before you start squeezing, take a look at some of the options.

Professional Extraction

The best thing you can do is see a skin specialist. A dermatologist or an esthetician can drain the pimple or blackhead. They're trained to know exactly how to treat a blemish without causing damage to the skin.

Extractions work especially well for blackheads. The pros can get rid of most of the existing blackheads on your skin in just a few visits.

Of course, it's not realistic to run to the skin doctor or salon every time a blemish appears. Both the cost and the time it takes are not likely to be practical.

If you have a pustule with a large, obvious white head, you can try a warm compress. Soak a soft cloth in warm water and hold it over the pimple for several minutes. Rewarm the compress when it gets cold.

The warmth helps to make the pore loose and open. It softens the pimple head and allows it to drain naturally. Don't do this until the pustule head is at the very surface of the skin. If you do this before it's ready, a pimple that's not quite formed will just get inflamed, look larger, and be more obvious.

The warm compress method won't work on blackheads. This is because the core of a blackhead is more hard and sticky than the core of a pustule.

Spot Treatment

If you have a day or so to wait, over-the-counter spot treatments are another good option. Dab a small amount on the pimple and leave it alone. The spot treatment helps dry up the pimple.

Hydrocolloid acne patches may help too. They'll keep you from picking at the pimple as it heals. You can get spot treatments in the skincare aisle of your local drug store. Products that contain benzoyl peroxide or sulfur tend to work best on white-head pustules.

Some people also have good results with products containing salicylic acid or tea tree oil. You may want to try a few brands in order to find the one that works best for your skin. Besides popping, you can try other ways to remove a pimple. Warm compresses may work on a fully formed pimple with a white head, or pustule. Over-the-counter skin care products also can help.

Safer Steps to Pop a Pimple

Ideally, you'll be able to take care of your pimple without squeezing. Popping pimples should always be a last resort.

But, if you're going to pop a pimple, it's best to do it safely. Remember that when you squeeze a blemish, you can cause damage to your skin. This steps will at least reduce the chance of that happening.

This only works for pimples with large, obvious whiteheads. They need to be close to the skin surface.

• Wash your hands well with soap and water.

• Sanitize a needle or pin with rubbing alcohol.

• Gently prick only the very top of the whitehead with the tip of the needle. Do so on an angle that is parallel to the skin. Don't go so deep that you draw blood. If this hurts, either you're poking too deeply or the pimple isn't ready to treat yet.

• Wrap your fingers in tissue or cotton. Place your fingers on either side of the blemish.

• Gently pull away from the blemish. This motion is the opposite of squeezing. It will often work to drain the pimple without the risk of pushing any infected matter deeper into the skin.

• Stop here if it works. There's no need to squeeze at all. Cleanse the area with soap or facial wash, and apply a bit of toner or astringent.

If you still have the whitehead:

• Grab two cotton swabs. Apply gentle pressure to the sides of the blemish. This is a better way to squeeze than using your fingers.

• Work the cotton swabs around the blemish. That way, you're not continually pushing from the same sides.

• Don't squeeze too hard or draw blood. You want just enough pressure to drain the whitehead.

• Once done, wash with cleanser. Apply toner or astringent. You can also use a tiny dab of antibacterial ointment on the pimple site.

Popping a pimple safely involves two main ideas. First, keep the site clean and sterile. Then, use only gentle pressure. Don't force it. If the pimple doesn't drain easily, then it's not ready. Leave it alone and try a spot treatment overnight.

Never Pop a Deep Inflamed Blemish

You can sometimes gently "pop" a whitehead. But there are certain types of pimples you should never try to pop. Don't do so if you see:

• Any red pimple without a white head

• Big, inflamed, deep blemishes. These may be nodular breakouts and cysts that should not be squeezed. The core is too deep in the skin, so it's best to simply let them heal on their own. A spot treatment or acne medication might help to get them on their way.

• A large and very painful blemish may not be a pimple. It may be a boil instead.

It's generally safer to extract a blackhead than an inflamed pimple. There is less risk of infection and scarring. Still, you'll need to treat your skin gently.

You may want to try removing a blackhead right after your shower or bath. The steam and warmth will relax the pore openings. This loosens and softens the blackhead plugs. It makes them easier to coax from the pore.

• Wash your hands with soap.

• Wrap your fingers in cotton or tissue.

• Place gentle pressure on either side of the blackhead. Try to get below the blackhead and push up carefully.

• Instead of steady pressure, massage the plug or use a rocking motion to help loosen it. Do this until the core is completely removed. Remember, don't press so hard that you draw blood or leave finger marks on your skin.

• Use a toner or astringent on all the areas that you've extracted.

Comedone Extractors

Comedone extractors are small metal tools estheticians use to remove blackheads. They can be an option. However, they also can do more harm than good in unskilled hands. It's easy to apply too much pressure and bruise your skin.

If you do use a comedone extractor, make sure you sanitize it first with rubbing alcohol. Put the loop of the tool around the blackhead, with the blackhead in the middle. Apply gentle pressure straight down, and don't dig into the skin. If you leave red marks on the skin, you're pushing too hard.

Some blemishes, like a red or inflamed one, should be left alone. Blackheads, though, may be easier to remove. You can do so by hand or, if you can use one safely, try the comedone extractor. Blackheads can be stubborn. If you can't extract them, leave them alone for another day.

DO ANTI-ACNE DIETS WORK?

There is so much information out there about acne and diet. Some experts claim certain foods can cause acne, and cutting those foods from your diet can improve acne. Others say there is no link between food and acne—that diet has nothing to do with the health of your skin.

Refined Carbohydrates

Not all carbs are equal and, according to a few studies, the wrong types could have an effect on your skin.

Researchers have found that high glycemic index foods (think white bread, potatoes, and sugary junk foods) seem to make acne worse. A diet rich in low glycemic index foods, which includes wheat bread, wheat pasta, legumes, and other whole grains, seems to improve acne. Much more research needs to be done though, as the info we have is still preliminary.

This sweet treat has been blamed for many a case of acne. How many of us have been warned to stay away from chocolate if we want clear skin?

Good news for all you chocoholics out there: chocolate does not cause acne. In fact, more data is coming out showing that chocolate (the darker the better) is actually good for you. Dark chocolate is full of healthful antioxidants.

Fried Foods

Does eating oily foods translate to oily skin? Chalk this one up as another acne-causes myth.

There are no way to disguise French fries, fried chicken, and other deep-fried morsels as health food, but they don't make your skin more oily. They won't make acne worse either.

For some people, dairy products may actually worsen acne. Several studies have shown a link between acne severity and consumption of milk and other dairy products.

It's still a stretch to say that milk causes acne, and giving up all dairy probably won't cause acne to disappear. Still, if you're a big milk drinker, you may want to cut back on the dairy for a while and see if it has any effect on your skin.

Organic Diet

Those organic grapes, tomatoes, and apples are amazingly tasty. And it's fun to browse the farmer's market for new and unique organic fare.

But will loading your diet with organic foods help to clear your skin? While there are many different reasons to go organic, clearing up acne isn't one of them.

No matter what some organic proponents say, the research just doesn't back this up. Eating organic foods may reduce the amount of pesticides you take in, but there is no indication that it has any effect on acne breakouts.

So, if the price of organic food gives you sticker shock, forgoing it for regular produce won't hurt your skin.

Sugar

While some people swear eating sugary foods makes their acne worse, the research linking sugar to acne development is pretty weak.

A handful of small studies suggest there may be a link, detractors are quick to point out that the pool of participants was quite small. Also, they relied on participants self-reporting acne breakouts—not a very objective way to classify changes in the skin.

From the information we have right now, it seems sugar doesn't play any role in acne development.

Interestingly, a diet rich in meat may raise your chances of developing acne through a complex chain reaction.

There is a protein-complex within the human body that some researchers believe is responsible for turning on this chain reaction that stimulates the skin's oil glands and makes acne breakouts more likely to develop. The trigger to get this process started is the amino acid leucine.

Foods like beef and chicken are naturally high in leucine. So far, there isn't any definitive proof, as this is just a theory. But it is an interesting look at how the skin works.

We do know, though, that acne development is very complex and it's highly unlikely that just changing one aspect of your diet is going to completely clear up a case of acne. Your best bet for treatment is still a proven acne medication.

CHAPTER FOUR

HOW TO REMOVE PIMPLE MARKS IN 12 EFFECTIVE WAYS

Pimple marks can be a cruel reminder of our skin woes. The best way to ignore getting pimples is by preventing breakouts and a balanced diet. However, there's much more than just a diet and lifestyle that contribute to pimple marks. These pesky pimple marks can really affect your confidence. But, there are more than one ways to know how to remove pimple marks.

What Causes Pimple Marks

Many people mistake acne and pimple as the same thing. While acne is a skin condition, pimples are a side effect of one of the symptoms of acne. Oily skin is one of the most affected skin types due to acne and pimples. The pimples and pimple spots appear, in most cases, as the natural boil on your skin. When your skin cells accumulate dirt, toxins and oil sebum, it leads to clogging of pores. This clogged pores, as result, lead to breakouts and pimples. To know how to remove pimple marks effectively, it is essential that you keep your face clean. Many people suffer from pimples due to hormonal changes. However, no matter what the case is, pimple marks are a dreaded nightmare for all of us.

Types Of Pimple Marks

There are primarily three types of pimple marks. They are usually identified by their appearance on the skin.

• Tiny ones that become flat and black-ish: These ones are the easiest to clear and often the process is natural.

• One with the white head: This one tends to scar the sin at a deeper level. Also called the ice pick, boxcar and rolling scars, these kinds of pimple marks look narrower, but have a deep effect. These marks are also due to collagen loss of the skin.

• Ones that leave red-brown-ish marks: These scars are caused by the cyst and hormonal imbalance, and are often very difficult to leave.

1. Orange Peel Powder

Full of the goodness of citric acid that helps in lightening the marks and brightening the skin, orange peel powder is a blessing for those who don't know how to remove pimple marks from their skin.

You Will Need

- 1 tsp orange peel powder

- 1 tsp raw honey

What To Do

1. Mix equal portions of orange peel powder with honey. Mix it well to remove all lumps and to make a smooth paste.

2. Apply this paste on affected areas of your face which are marred by pimples.

3. Let it stay for 10-15 minutes and wash it off with lukewarm water.

Tip: Try this once every alternate day to remove pimple marks.

2. Coconut Oil

There's hardly any skin condition that can't benefit from the rich, anti-inflammatory and anti-bacterial properties of coconut oil. This effective home remedy is a sure-shot way to prevent the surfacing of new acne lesions. Packed with vitamins E and K, and antioxidants, it helps in the growth of healthy skin cells that helps to remove pimple marks.

You Will Need

• 1 tsp coconut oil

What To Do

1. Rub coconut oil between your palms and dab it gently over affected areas of your face

2. Leave it overnight for a better result, and wash

Tip: Try this daily to see better results.

3. Besan

Being one of the most easily available ingredients, besan (gram flour) comes in handy for most skin troubles. Be it to remove pimple marks or to be used as a regular face scrub, besan is full of alkalizing properties, and it has been used as a skin cleanser for years to maintain the skin's pH balance.

You Will Need

• 1 tbsp of besan

• Rosewater

• Lemon juice

What To Do

1. Mix besan, rose water and lemon juice to make a paste of thick texture.

2. Apply the paste evenly on your face and neck, especially concentrate more on the affected areas.

3. Let it dry and wash with plain water.

Tips: Do it every alternate day for better results. You can also eliminate lemon juice from the process if you like.

4. Tea Tree Oil

For acne and pimple-prone skin, tea tree oil is a savior. Its anti-inflammatory and antimicrobial properties play a perfect agent to get rid of marks and blemishes on the skin. The best part of this home remedy is that it works well for every skin type.

You Will Need

• Three to four drops of tea tree oil

• Carrier oil like coconut or almond oil

What To Do

1. Mix tea tree oil with a carrier oil

2. Mix it well to make a paste and apply it uniformly to the pimple marks and lesions.

3. Let it stay overnight or for at least one or two hours before washing it off.

Tips: Try this daily for best results. Since tea tree oil needs a carrier oil, you can use any essential or mineral oil instead of coconut oil.

5. Apple Cider Vinegar

If you want to strike the perfect pH balance for your sin, apple cider vinegar is an effective ingredient. It soaks in excess oils and keeps the skin pores clean and exfoliated naturally, leaving soft, smooth and blemishes-free skin. It also helps in reducing the redness of your pimples, and gradually helps in the reduction of their size.

You Will Need

• 1 tbsp apple cider vinegar

• 2 tbsps honey

• Water

What To Do

• Mix apple cider vinegar with two tbsps of honey.

• Use water if you want to dilute the consistency of this mixture.

• Apply this mixture on your entire face using a clean cotton pad.

• Let it stay for 15 to 20 minutes and wash with plain water.

Tips: Try this daily for effective results. If you have sensitive skin, dilute mix one part apple cider vinegar with 10 parts water.

6. Aloe Vera

For flawless, naturally-glowing skin, aloe vera is a perfect remedy. With its antioxidant and anti-inflammatory properties, it helps in curing skin woes like scars, pimple marks, and infections. It also relieves the skin of blemishes and aids in healing wounds faster without leaving marks.

You Will Need

• Aloe vera gel

What To Do

1. Extract the gel from aloe leaves or buy organic aloe vera gel or gel-based products from the market.

2. Apply a thick and uniform layer to the affected area.

3. Leave it on your face staying overnight.

Tips: Try this daily. With its multiple health benefits, you can apply this to your hair, body and face. You can also drink it to enhance your skin pH balance.

7. Baking Soda

Baking soda is known for its exfoliating and bleaching properties. Regularly use of baking soda helps in getting rid of clogged skin pores and skin marks. Owing to its alkaline nature, this ingredient also helps in restoring the skin's pH balance pH and aids in combatting scars and pimple.

You Will Need

• 2 tbsps baking soda

• 1 tbsp water

What To Do

1. Take water and baking soda in a small bowl. Mix well and apply it on your scars.

2. Let it dry and wash it off after 10-12 minutes

Tips: Try this once a day. Please ensure that you're using baking soda and not baking powder.

8. Lemon Juice

Lemon juice is a natural bleaching agent. With its lightening properties, it can be used to lighten the pimple marks easily.

You Will Need

• Fresh lemon juice

• Cotton pads

What To Do

1. Take the lemon juice and rub it gently on your pimple marks and other affected areas. Squeeze the juice from half a lemon.

2. You can use a cotton pad or your fingers. Make sure your hands are clean.

3. Let it rest for 10-15 minutes. Wash with lukewarm water.

Tips: Do it every alternate day. Use fresh lemons for effective results. You must do this once every alternate day.

9. Castor Oil

Castor oil contains vitamin E and omega-3 fatty acids. These enriching elements help in repairing the damaged skin layer by helping in the growth of new skin cells. It also helps in fighting pigmentation, reduces the size of the acne scars.

You Will Need

• Castor oil (as required)

What To Do

1. Take some oil on your fingers and apply it to the affected areas.

2. Leave it on overnight and wash off the next morning with lukewarm water.

Tips: Since castor oil has a thick consistency, it is imperative that you make sure it has completely washed away.

10. Turmeric

Turmeric is perhaps one of the oldest medicinal herbs that humans know. Its anti-inflammatory and antioxidant properties speed up and lighten acne scars and skin tone. Regular use of turmeric powder on the skin aids in the reduction of pigmentation and also gives a glowing skin tone.

You Will Need

• 1-2 tsp of turmeric powder

• 1 spoon lemon juice

What To Do

1. Mix turmeric powder and lemon juice.

2. Apply this paste evenly all over your face like a face mask

3. Leave it on your skin for 30 minutes

4. Wash it off with lukewarm water

Tips: You must do this once every alternate day. If you don't want your fingers stained yellow, wear gloves when applying the mask, as it leaves a yellowish tint on the skin.

11. Shea Butter

Shea Butter contains anti-inflammatory properties by virtue of it having Vitamin F and other such healthy fatty acids. These elements serve the purpose of reducing inflammation around the scars and injecting moisture into them, which weakens the appearance of said pimple or acne scars.

You Will Need

• 1 tablespoon of raw shea butter

• 5 drops of lavender essential oil

• 3 drops of lemon essential oil

What To Do

1. Put a tablespoon of raw shea butter in a medium-sized bowl.

2. Use a whisk to stir the shea butter until it becomes creamy.

3. Add the essential oils and continue stirring

Tips: Apply the shea butter every night for best results.

12. Potato

This is one of the best methods to get rid of those pesky acne and pimple scars and return your natural glow. This is possible as potatoes are rich and vitamins and minerals that only help remove scars but can also help remove blackheads and excess oil from your face.

You Will Need

• A Potato

What To Do

• Rub a potato slice onto the affected area

• Leave the juice on your face for 15-20 minutes

• Rinse it off with water

• Repeat once daily until you get the results

Tips: You can eat potatoes to have better skin as well, however, the benefits are limited to the way you choose to cook the potatoes. Avoid frying them!

Prevention Tips Pimple Marks

• Keep your face clean and wash it at least twice a day with a milder face wash.

• Exfoliate regularly. It helps your skin to get rid of dead skin cells and helps in keeping the pores clean.

• Never go to bed with makeup on.

• Use chemical-free makeup remover. Use clean cotton pads to remove makeup, as it often ends up leading the pores to clog.

• If you are suffering from a breakout, never touch or pop any pimple.

• Keep away from direct sun. Always wear sunscreen if you spend a lot of time outdoors.

• A healthy diet is the best way to keep breakouts. Eat a lot of greens and drink plenty of healthy fluids for natural skin.

Tips: These home remedies can solve most of your skin woes. However, some serious skin conditions need a dermatologist's opinion. If your pimples or acne don't go away after two weeks, do see a skin specialist. This could also be hormonal. Some scar marks do not fade away with time. They surely do lighten up, but never go away completely. If you are suffering from such a skin condition, take a dermatologist's opinion on pimple marks.

HOW OFTEN YOU SHOULD WASH YOUR FACE IF YOU HAVE ACNE

Acne isn't caused by neglecting to wash your face. Other factors, like bacteria or changing hormones, cause this skin condition. Yet regular cleansing is a key step in your acne treatment routine.

There is such a thing as getting your skin "too clean," though. If you wonder how many times a day you should wash your face, the magic number is generally agreed to be two.

Twice-Daily Washing

If you wash your face in the morning and at night, it will be enough to clean away makeup, dirt, and the extra oil on your skin that can contribute to breakouts.

What you use to cleanse your face also matters. The skin on your face is delicate, so you don't want to use harsh soaps. Antibacterial hand soap and bar soaps are unsuitable for your skin if you have acne. It would help if you never used rubbing alcohol on your face either.

Stronger isn't always better. Instead, choose a cleanser that leaves your skin feeling clean but not overly dry or stripped.

Acne Isn't Caused by a Dirty Face

If you're prone to breaking out, it's important to know that it doesn't mean you aren't taking proper care of your skin.

People with acne has skin cells that don't shed away correctly. They are more sensitive to irritation caused by Propionibacteria acnes, an acne-causing bacteria.

Hormones play a role in whether you develop acne, too. Acne is caused by factors like bacteria and hormones — not a dirty face. Still, you should remove dirt and oil by washing your face morning and night with a gentle cleanser.

Washing your face too much can be just as bad (or even worse) than not doing it at all. Scrubbing hard is to be avoided too. You can easily strip away all of the good oils your skin needs to stay healthy, leaving you with dry, red, flaky, and irritated skin.

You can also break down the acid mantle. This is a protective layer on the skin made up of sweat, oil, and good bacteria. Healthy skin needs a strong, healthy acid mantle.

One exception to this? A third cleansing in a day is recommended if you get particularly sweaty or dirty.

Cleansing Alone Isn't Enough for Acne

Good skin care means removing dirt, excess oil, and makeup. It can help to keep your pores from being plugged up. Still, water and a simple soap or face wash aren't enough to clear up acne.

Think of your twice-daily cleansing as a first step in treating your acne. Step two should be the routine use of an acne treatment product.

For mild breakouts, you might try over-the-counter acne products first. The most effective products contain salicylic acid and benzoyl peroxide.

Try to use them regularly for a few weeks to see if that helps clear things up. Facial scrubs also may help. Some of the available product brands, and their various formulas, include:

• Proactive

• Benzaderm Gel

• Neutrogena

• PanOxyl

• Noxzema

• Oxy

• Stridex

Harsh scrubs won't clear your skin faster, but they can irritate it and make breakouts worse. Remember that all acne medications that go on your skin, whether over-the-counter or prescription, work best when applied to freshly washed and thoroughly dried skin.

More severe or inflamed bouts with acne usually don't get better with a store-bought acne product. Instead, you'll need a prescription acne medication from your healthcare provider. These treatments include Differin (adapalene), Retin-A (tretinoin), and Tazorac (tazarotene).

Cleansing your face more than twice daily can irritate and degrade your skin's natural protective layer. Wash your face as advised, then follow up with an OTC or prescription acne treatment.

CHAPTER FIVE

6 STEPS TO HEALTHIER SKIN

A good daily skin care routine is important for everyone, but especially so when you're prone to acne. These six steps will help you create happy, healthy skin and control breakouts, too.

Cleansing

The backbone of your skin care routine has to be good cleansing. Thorough cleansing keeps the skin free of excess oil, dirt, sweat, and makeup, and leaves a nice, clean base for your acne treatment products.

But good cleansing goes beyond just soap and water. First, you have to start off with the right cleanser for your skin—nothing too harsh or drying. Antibacterial soaps aren't a good choice for just this reason.

For most people, a twice-daily cleansing is a good goal. Don't forget to wash your face before bed.

Exfoliation

In order to fight acne, you need to hit it where it starts —
in the pore. Regular exfoliation helps to keep the pores
free of excess skin cells and oil. Exfoliation removes dead
skin cell buildup, reduces the formation of comedones,
and helps smooth and soften the skin.

Grainy face and body scrubs immediately come to mind,
but they might not be the best exfoliating products for
acne-prone skin. Scrubs can irritate the skin if you're not
using them gently.

You might not need a separate exfoliating product,
though. Many acne treatment products, both over-the-
counter and prescription, have exfoliating properties
already.

Toning

Toners and astringents are used after cleansing, to leave
your skin feeling fresh. Astringents are specially
designed to remove extra oil from the skin. Some also
contain blemish-fighting ingredients like salicylic acid.

But these aren't a necessary part of your daily skin care routine. Deciding to use an astringent, or not, depends on many factors. If your skin is sensitive, dry, or irritated from your acne treatments, toners and astringents may do more harm than good.

Moisturizing

Many people with oily skin steer clear of moisturizers. But moisturizing is a good thing, even if you're acne-prone.

A good, oil-free moisturizer won't trigger breakouts, but will help ease dryness, flakiness, and peeling. Acne treatments can completely dry out your skin and you will want moisturizing to counteract that.

The trick Is choosing the right moisturizer for your blemish-prone skin. One that is labeled oil-free and noncomedogenic is your best bet.

Your skin needs to be protected from the sun. Sunscreen prevents more than just sunburn; it reduces your chance of developing premature lines and wrinkles, dark spots, and skin cancer.

There are plenty of good sunscreens out there today that aren't heavy or greasy, and won't clog your pores and make acne worse. Since many acne medications make your skin more sensitive to the sun, wearing sunscreen daily is extra important for good skin health.

And don't think sunscreen is just for summertime skin care. Dermatologists recommend wearing sunscreen year-round for the best protection. That means your wintertime skin care routine should include sunscreen too.

Daily Acne Treatment Medication

Your skin care regimen doesn't have to take a lot of time, just a few minutes twice a day. To really clear up acne, though, good skin care is just one piece of the puzzle.

Controlling acne relies on a two-pronged approach—a consistent daily skin care routine plus effective acne treatment medications.

Acne medications help clear up existing breakouts while keeping new blemishes from forming. Over-the-counter acne treatments can help with milder forms of acne. Stubborn cases will need a prescription acne medication.

Your dermatologist can get you the right acne treatment for your skin, and help you create the right skin care regimen for you.

EXFOLIATION TIPS TO HELP ACNE-PRONE SKIN

If you're interested in skincare, you probably have already heard the term exfoliation. Exfoliation is beneficial for all skin types, but especially so for acne-prone skin. But what exactly is exfoliation? (Hint: it's not just about a scrub.)

In simple terms, exfoliation is the removal of dead skin cells. An exfoliant is a product or procedure that reduces the amount of dead cell build-up on the skin.

Your skin naturally exfoliates, or sheds dead cells, through a process called desquamation. But in people with acne, this natural process isn't working as effectively as it should.

Dead skin cells are hanging around longer than they should, plugging up the pores and creating comedones. All pimples begin as comedones.

Whether your acne is mild or more severe, regular exfoliation will smooth and soften the skin and brighten your complexion. It also helps reduce breakouts by keeping the pores from becoming clogged with the pus of dead cells and sebum (skin oil).

But before you run out and buy an abrasive scrub, take the time to learn about all the exfoliating products and treatments available. Making the right exfoliant choice is essential for getting good results without irritating your skin and aggravating acne.

There are literally hundreds of exfoliating products and procedures available today, but all are found in one of two forms: physical or chemical.

Physical Exfoliants

You're probably most familiar with physical exfoliants. Physical exfoliants manually remove dead skin cells by use of an abrasive ingredient or implement. Gritty scrubs, rough cleansing pads and cloths, and professional microdermabrasion procedures are all examples of physical exfoliants.

Physical exfoliants leave your skin feeling soft and smooth, but they often aren't the best exfoliant choice for acne-prone skin. The friction involved in using a physical exfoliant can irritate already inflamed skin.

This rubbing and scrubbing can leave your skin looking redder and can make existing breakouts worse by irritating and exacerbating redness. The more inflamed your acne, the more you'll want to avoid physical exfoliants.

If you have inflammatory acne, you should avoid physical exfoliants altogether unless otherwise advised by your healthcare provider.

Chemical Exfoliants

Chemical exfoliants work without abrasive agents. Instead, chemical exfoliants dissolve or loosen the bonds that hold dead cells on the skin's surface by means of an acid or enzyme.

Even if you weren't familiar with the term "chemical exfoliant," you're probably familiar with the products or procedures. You've most likely used some before too.

Some common chemical exfoliants include:

• Alpha hydroxy acids (AHA) like glycolic, lactic, and tartaric acid

• Beta hydroxy acids (BHA) like salicylic acid

• Topical retinoids, including Differin (adapalene), retinol and Retin-A (tretinoin)

• Chemical peels, from superficial chemical peels to deeper trichloroacetic acid (TCA), carbolic or phenol peels

Over-the-counter chemical exfoliants can be found at your local retail store, and many are gentle enough to be used daily. OTC glycolic peels, for example, are very popular at-home chemical exfoliants.

Stronger treatments, like salicylic acid peels, are available at day spas and skin spas. The estheticians working there can help you decide which treatments will be best for your skin.

For the most powerful chemical exfoliant products, ask your dermatologist. He or she can provide you with a prescription medication like topical retinoids, or perform stronger chemical peels if needed.

Most chemical exfoliants, whether over-the-counter or healthcare provider prescribed, will dry the skin to some degree. Incorporating an oil-free moisturizer into your daily skin care routine will help ward off excessive dryness, peeling, and irritation.

Exfoliating Safety Tips

If you need help choosing an exfoliant, don't hesitate to ask your dermatologist for guidance. Your healthcare provider will be able to recommend a product or procedure that is both safe and effective for your skin.

Unless recommended by your healthcare provider, avoid using several exfoliating products at the same time. Doing so may cause redness, excessive dryness, peeling, and considerable irritation. Remember, too much of a good thing is too much.

Exfoliation is a beneficial part of any skincare routine. With regular exfoliation your skin will look brighter, and feel softer and smoother. It can also help clear out your pores, and reduce breakouts. Some exfoliating products can help improve signs of aging too.

If you are currently using any acne medications, especially isotretinoin or topical retinoids, talk with your healthcare provider before beginning any exfoliation treatment. In fact, if you're seeing a healthcare provider for any skin issue, you should get her OK before making any changes to your skincare routine.

CONCLUSION

There are four main types of pimples. These include papules, pustules, nodules, and cysts. Papules and pustules can be treated at home. Try a benzoyl peroxide cleanser or a salicylic spot treatment.

Nodules and acne cysts may require help from a dermatologist. A dermatologist can give you a cortisone injection or prescribe medication that will help clear up your skin.

Getting a pimple every now and again isn't a big deal. If you're constantly battling breakouts and struggling to get them under control, though, it's time to make an appointment with a dermatologist. This is especially true if you're prone to larger blemishes like acne nodules. Medications can help you clear your skin.

Everyone gets pimples, whether occasionally or on a more consistent basis. Although nothing can heal a pimple instantaneously, or even overnight, the above tips can help speed healing, or at least make the blemish look and feel better while it does.

If your pimple is especially large or painful or isn't healing, you should call your healthcare provider. Your blemish may need to be surgically excised (AKA acne surgery). It also may not be an acne pimple at all but possibly another acne-like skin condition, like a boil or epidermoid cyst.

The best way to treat pimple is to stop them before they even start by using proven acne treatments regularly. See a dermatologist if you need help. They'll be happy to share their acne treatment secrets with you to get your blemishes under control.